# THE FRENCH PARADOX

**The French are protected by their diet.
They have:
- fewer cardiovascular diseases
- a weapon against ageing.**

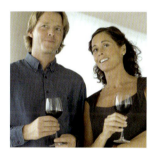

Isabelle Brette

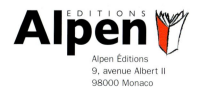
EDITIONS
Alpen

Alpen Éditions
9, avenue Albert II
98000 Monaco

**Exclusive copyrights:**
©Alpen Éditions
9, avenue Albert II
98000 Monaco
Tel: +377 97 77 62 10
Fax: +377 97 77 62 11
web: www.alpen.mc


Printed in Italy
ISBN: 978-2-35934-041-9

# THE FRENCH PARADOX

**The French are protected by their diet.**
**They have:**
**- fewer cardiovascular diseases**
**- a weapon against ageing.**

*It's natural, it's my health*

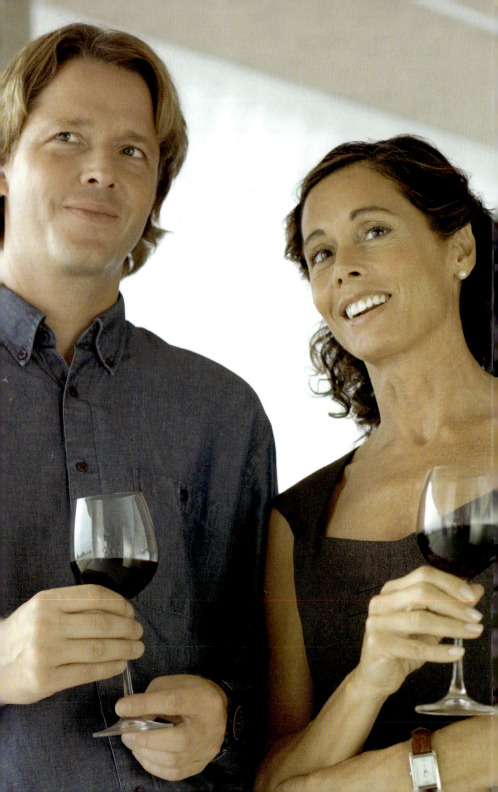

# Introduction

## Eating fruits and vegetables and drinking wine to live better and longer. What is the French secret?

The French have the reputation for enjoying both eating and drinking. Yet, on average they die less from coronary heart diseases than others. In addition, their consumption of saturated fats, that contribute to bad cholesterol (called LDL cholesterol), is practically the same as elsewhere. So what is their secret?

One of the keys to French diet is wine. Many studies have shown that there is a correlation between the quantity of wine (mainly red) that they drink every day and the rate of cardiovascular events. This is the famous French paradox, a concept that originated around 20 years ago, which promotes wine as a major health asset, as long as it is drunk in moderation. Studies have shown that 1 to 2 glasses of red wine per day can decrease the risk of heart attacks.

Wine owes its beneficial properties to polyphenols, compounds found in significant quantities in the solid parts of grapes (skin and seeds). The polyphenols (also known as antioxidants) protect blood vessel walls, decrease their permeability and due to their antioxidising action, help manage blood cholesterol levels. But there is more: red wine continues to surprise us. Over time wine has revealed other health benefits. When drunk in moderation, it may have an anti-ageing power that slows the process of skin ageing. This is also thanks to its high concentration of polyphenols, those formidable natural antioxidants. By destroying free radicals, they contribute to preserving collagen in the skin whose production starts to naturally decrease from age 20.

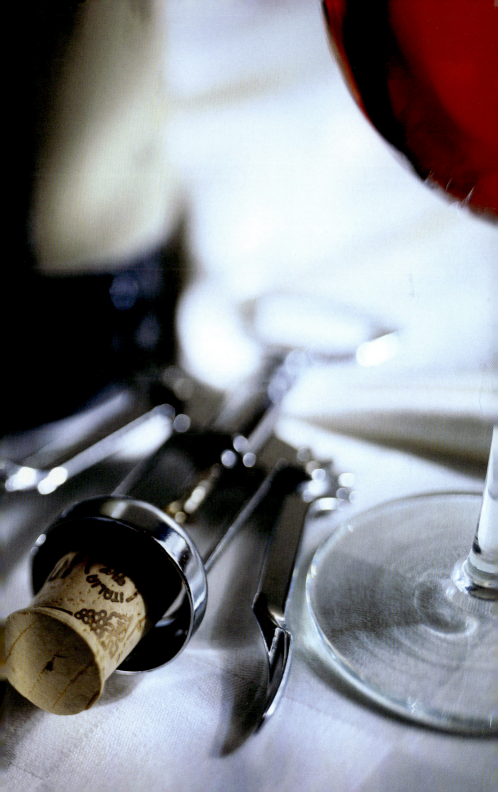

# TABLE OF CONTENTS

# AN IDENTITY INHERITED FROM THE ROMANS

**What is there in the French diet that protects them more than others against cardio-vascular diseases? Why do they (along with the Japanese) have one of the longest life expectancies on the planet? Answer: they eat plenty of fruits and vegetables, and drink one to two glasses of red wine per day.**

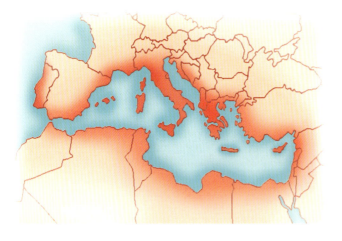

It is impossible to run out of good things to say about the French diet. Despite a high consumption of saturated fats in the form of butter, cheese, cream, eggs and fatty and processed meats, the French have a lower rate of cardiovascular diseases than elsewhere in the world: On the other side of the Atlantic, there are 320 heart attacks per 100,000 middle aged inhabitants compared to 145 in France. The secret of the French, just like it has long been of the Cretans in Greece, is their daily consumption of fruits and vegetables, plus one or two glasses of red wine.

# THE MEDITERRANEAN DIET

## Thanks to the Romans

The area around the Mediterranean is a vast garden where grapes grow in abundance, and where the trees bend under fruit bursting with goodness. It is a garden of colours and flavours. But it wasn't always like this and we are in debt to the Romans for this. Their Mediterranean empire encouraged trading between cultures. Thanks to them olive oil spread throughout the basin and they founded a culture of grapes, fruits, certain vegetables and grains from newly conquered regions. This sharing of produce made it possible to create original, highly diversified dishes.

## A vitamin cocktail

Question: What do the lemon, kiwi, orange, grapefruit, papaya, tangerine, strawberry, rockmelon,and green and red vegetables all have in common?
*They are rich sources of vitamins including vitamin C, vitamin E and beta carotene (precursor of vitamin A).*

Question: What do all the foods of the plant kingdom have in common?
*They contain phytonutrients, including polyphenols, as well as tannins and flavonoids.*

Question: What do vitamins and polyphenols have in common?
*They are strong antioxidants.*

The answers above provide an entry point to begin explaining the French paradox and its benefits on our health.

## History of the Mediterranean diet

The Mediterranean diet originated thousands of years ago. It is based on the consumption of cereals, vegetables and legumes, dairy products and fruit. It is often represented in the form of a pyramid, with the base composed of foods to be eaten regularly in large quantities (cereals, fruit, vegetables and wine in moderation) and at the top those which should only be eaten occasionally (fatty meats, cold cuts, sweets, etc.).

# Characteristics

**Diet plays a major role in our health. Too many kilojoules, too much saturated fat, too much sugar, and too few fruits, vegetables and fibre are major contributors for many chronic diseases such as obesity, diabetes and cardiovascular diseases.**

Various studies conducted around the world have shown that the Mediterranean diet makes it possible to decrease morbidity and mortality from cardiovascular diseases. And it is not just a question of intake, but also a philosophy: The Mediterranean diet is a true way of living and in that sense it is associated with the idea of pleasure and socialising. It takes into account the time it takes to eat which helps with adequate chewing and digestion. It is completely the opposite of the fast-food concept long considered as a model by many western countries (we now know how bad this is for you). The last, but not least important component of the diet in question, is physical activity. We need to remember that our hunter-gatherer ancestors had to walk kilometres to find food, and they did not suffer from high blood pressure and obesity.

## The Mediterranean diet: what is it?

The Mediterranean diet compromises of:
• Cereals: wholegrain and bread (whole wheat since it is richer in fibre).
• Vegetables and fruits, nuts and seeds. These are good sources of fibre, vitamins, minerals and antioxidants. Current nutrition guidelines recommend consuming at least 5 serves of vegetables and 2 of fruits each day for good health.

• Dairy products mainly in the form of yoghurt and cheese are ideal for calcium needs, but otherwise the Mediterranean diet contains very little butter and milk which are full of saturated fats.
• Olive oil, a rich source of mono-unsaturated fat.
• Small amounts of meat (lamb, veal and pork).
• Fish: rich in omega-3 fatty acids shown to help reduce the risk of cardiovascular disease.

This diet also includes wine in moderate amounts. In small quantities alcohol can increase good cholesterol (HDL). Red wine also has the protective benefit of polyphenols and in particular from flavonoids where tannins are found.

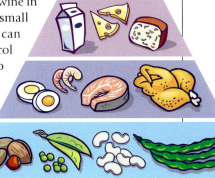
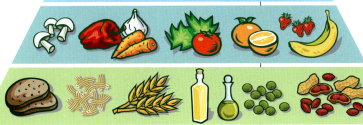

**The Mediterranean food pyramid**

# Full of vitamins

**We need vitamins to live. However, they are not a direct source of energy, nor do they make up our tissue, but if they are lacking, nutrients like carbohydrates, fats and proteins will not be used effectively by our boby.**

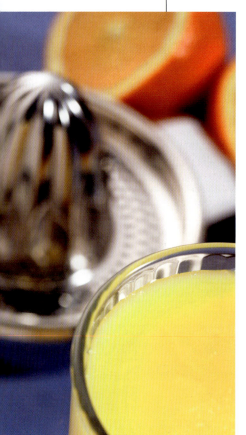

Vitamins are found in the food we eat. There are 13 vitamins : A, C, D, E, K and eight B vitamins: folic acid, thiamin (B1), riboflavin (B2), pantothenic acid (B5), pyridoxine (B6), cyanocobalamin (B12), niacin (B3) and biotin.

## Vitamin C

Vitamin C is undoubtedly the best know vitamin. For the general public it is known for its cold fighting powers. It actually has other virtues including its role as an antioxidant and as an anti ageing vitamin.
Where is it found? In fruits and vegetables. The main sources of vitamin C are green and red capsicum, kiwi fruit, strawberries, citrus fruit (oranges, lemons, grapefruits and tangerines), cauliflower, mangoes and spinach. Contrary to popular belief, the orange doesn't have the highest vitamin C content. By weight, it actually contains less than kiwi fruit and fresh parsley!

## Vitamin A

Essential for vision and bone development it is also a beauty aid since it prevents signs of ageing by helping with skin cell regeneration. Where is it found? In orange and yellow fruit and vegetables, as well as in milk, eggs and liver.

## Vitamin D

It plays an essential role in bone mineralisation. Around two thirds of our vitamin D requirements come from the sun. Exposure to sunlight effectively contributes to its synthesis in the deep skin layers. The remaining third must come from our diet. Its main sources are fish, eggs and margarine enriched with vitamin D.

## Vitamin E

Helps decrease bad cholesterol, is important for blood circulation and decreases the risks of cardiovascular diseases. It also helps keep the immune system healthy. Where is it found? In walnuts, grains, oil (olive, peanut and sunflower) and in fruits and vegetables.

## Sources of Vitamin C

The amount of vitamin C in a range of different foods (per 100g) is shown below:

| | | | |
|---|---|---|---|
| Oranges | 58mg | Paw Paw | 60mg |
| Strawberries | 45mg | Parsley | 132mg |
| Kiwifruit | 71mg | Cherry tomato | 28mg |
| Red capsicum | 152mg | Cauliflower | 67mg |
| Mandarin | 58mg | | |

*Source: NUTTAB Nutrient Data for Australian Foods 2006*

### Vitamin K

It is essential for healthy blood clotting. In healthy people, the bacteria in the intestine normally supply a significant quantity of vitamin K.

Where is it found? In green leafy vegetables, liver, broad beans, soy, egg yolk, wheat, oatmeal, potatoes, asparagus and cheese.

### Vitamin B

Our bodies get great benefits from B vitamins. They are essential for metabolism (B1, B2, B3, B6, biotin and pantothenic acid), immune and nerve functions (B1, B6, folic acid, biotin and pantothenic acid) help keep skin healthy (B2 and biotin) and build strong muscles (B1). They are excellent for stress and help reduce the risk of cardiovascular diseases (B6, B12 and folic acid). Where are they found?

B1: wholegrain cereals, wheat germ, seeds, legumes, watermelon, yeast and pork. In Australia, flour is also fortified with thiamin.

B2: milk, yoghurt, cottage cheese, wholegrain breads & cereals, eggs, leafy green vegetables and meat.

B3: lean meats, wholegrain breads & cereals, milk, eggs, nuts and green leafy vegetables.

B6: grains, legumes, green leafy vegetables, fruit, fish, shellfish, meat & poultry, nuts and liver.

B12: kidney, liver, seafood, sardines, salmon and egg yolk.

B9 (folic acid): leafy green vegetables (eg. lettuce and

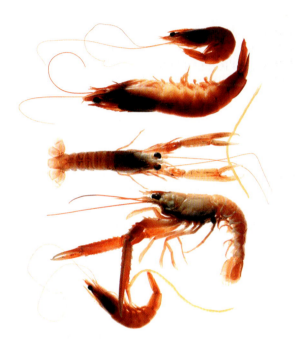

spinach) yeast, liver, broad beans, peanuts, almonds, strawberries, whole-wheat bread and folate fortified cereals.

Biotin: cauliflower, egg yolks, peanuts, liver, chicken, yeast and mushrooms.

Pantothenic acid: yeast, liver, kidney, eggs, peanut products, rice and wheat bran.

# POLYPHENOLS

# What are antioxidants?

**Antioxidants work to fight against the free radicals that are constantly produced by our bodies or formed as a response to our environment (smoking, pollutants, etc.) Free radicals contribute to cell ageing.**

## A question of balance

Antioxidants work to fight against free radicals. Too many free radicals are bad for our health. There is a permanent balance between these chemicals in our bodies. Antioxidants act to eliminate excess free radicals. The problems occur when there is an imbalance. This can be linked to our diet (when there are not enough antioxidants in our food), or environmental factors such as those described above.

## Two lines of defense

Our body has various defences to protect itself against free radicals. The first is composed of three enzymes that ensure an effective protection system for proteins, fats and DNA.

They are backed by a second line of defence that comes from the outside. This comes from our food and when needed from antioxidants which are vitamins C and E, carotenoids or pro-vitamin A (beta carotene) and polyphenols. Associated with a Mediterranean diet, polyphenols are the most abundant antioxidants in our

## Did you know?

Polyphenols are the most plentiful antioxidant in our diet and represent 1 gram per day.

food and are found in fruits and vegetables. The main polyphenol found are flavonoids. The amount of flavonoids supplied through food (apples, vegetables, tea, cocoa and wine) is estimated to average between 20 to 30 mg in Western Europe.

## Our diet supplies us with ten times more polyphenols than vitamin C

Research has shown that antioxidants prevent oxidation caused by free radicals. But which polyphenols are the most effective antioxidants, vitamin C, vitamin E or carotenoids?

Answer: it all depends on quantity. Through food humans take in around one gram of polyphenols each day, which is ten times more than vitamin C and a hundred times more than carotenoids or vitamin E, and it is estimated that fruits and vegetables contribute to half of this intake.

## Mainly in fruit

Polyphenols are particularly plentiful in fruit. Their content can reach 500 mg per 100 grams in certain fruit like apples, grapes or cherries, even up to one gram with persimmons.

Their content is much lower in vegetables, around 25 to 100 mg per 100 grams.

A simple tip: to be sure you are filling up on polyphenols, look at the colour of the fruit.

Red skin fruits are one class of polyphenols while the anthocyanins or yellow fruits are another.

# Where are they found?

**Polyphenols are mainly found in plant foods. Long considered as compounds with no nutritional value, they became highlighted as a key aspect of the French paradox. The presence of polyphenols in fruits and vegetables and wine (mainly red) explains the surprising "resistance" the French have to coronary diseases.**

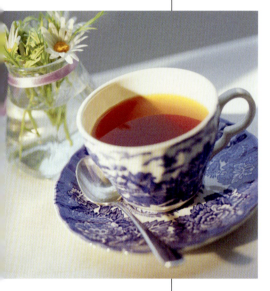

Polyphenols are mainly present in plant foods and are widely distributed in food, in particular in vegetables, fruit and legumes, where they contribute to the development of the colour and flavours. In general, a regular consumption of fruits and vegetables has a beneficial effect on health thanks to the polyphenols which are present in all the parts of the plant: roots, stems, flowers and leaves.

## Polyphenols – a large family
Polyphenols make up a large chemical family of more than 4000 compounds. They are divided into various classes, where the flavonoids are among the most important. Flavonoids are divided into various classes. The main flavonol is quercetin which is found in numerous fruits and vegetables and in wine. This substance is also particularly abundant in onions and tea. The main flavonols, better known as tannins, are mainly represented by catechins which are found in high quantities in tea and chocolate.
Proanthocyanines are also found in the flavonol family, primarily in purple and blue fruit (blueberries, cur-

| Isoflavons | Procyanidins (flavanol polymers) | Anthocyanins | Flavonols | Flavones | Flavanols | Flavanones |
|---|---|---|---|---|---|---|
| Soybeans | Fruits (pears, apples and grapes) | Red berries | Onions | Parsley | Apricots | Citrus fruits |
| Red clover leaves | Wines | Wines | Kale | Red pepper | Tea | |
| Barley | Tea | Grapes | Leek | Celery | Wines | |
| Brown rice | | Tea | Broccoli | Citrus fruits | Grapes | |
| Whole wheat | | | Blueberries | Onions | Chocolate | |
| Linseed | | | Wines | | Apples | |
| | | | Green teas | | | |
| | | | Tomatoes | | | |

rents, bilberries and black grapes) and red wines, and which give them their astringency, i.e. that rough sensation on the tongue when eating them.

There is also phloridzin, found in apples, zeaxanthine, cryptoxanthine, capsantol, capsorubin and capsanthin mainly present in young sprout and the above ground parts of lettuce, cabbage, spinach, broccoli and string beans and terpenes, primarily found in spices and herbs.

## Under the sun, even more polyphenols

The synthesis of flavonoids by the plant lets it protect itself from oxidation reactions. This explains why sunlight increases the quantity of flavonoids and why, in the same vegetable, the parts exposed to the sun have the highest contents.

# Antioxidants - Natural Protection

**Oligomeric procyanidins (OPC) are natural molecules found throughout nature. They are found in vegetables, fruits and cereals but also in grape seeds and pine bark. The nutritional and physiological interest in these molecules is linked to their antioxidant properties. They have a known effect on cardiovascular diseases.**

## Chemical structure

The OPC's belong to the polyphenol family and in particular to the class of flavonoids. They are polymers with the same molecular unit as catechin. In addition, they form the pigments responsible for the colour of fruits and vegetables.

## In the peel of fruits and vegetables.

OPC's are relatively plentiful in nature, but we get few from our diet. This is due to the fact that they are mainly present in the peels of fruits and vegetables, cuticles covering grape seeds or in grains: basically, in all the parts we reject in our diet.

## Antioxidant properties

The OPC's often end up in the bin with the peels. Too bad! Since these compounds have an antioxidant action 20 to 50 times higher than vitamins C and E. And unlike these vitamins which are water soluble (vitamin C) and fat soluble (vitamin E), the OPC's are both and thus protect cells from free radical attack two times better.

## Vascular protection

When blood vessels are in poor condition, blood has a hard time returning to the heart.

The legs become heavy and painfully swollen: this is typical of poor blood circulation. Thanks to their particular affinity with collagen (a protein which forms the essential part of connective tissues in the body), specifically the inner wall of blood vessels, the OPC's inhibit the action of certain collagen destructive enzymes, eg collagenases and thus help to keep the structure of these connective tissues intact. By helping the vein walls to maintain their elasticity and resistance, the OPC's have a beneficial action for circulation.

## Protection against skin ageing

The skin is also one of the connective tissues of the body. And just like vein walls, the skin also contains a significant quantity of collagen. By inhibiting the action of collagenases, OPC's help to reinforce the elasticity and suppleness of our skin.

## Why grape OPC's?

The history of OPC's dates back to Jacques Cartier. While en route to the New World in 1534, his ship got stuck in the ice of St. Lawrence river where it remained blocked for several weeks. The crew fell victim to scurvy, and was saved by Native Americans, thanks to teas made from pine needles and bark. At that time the disease killed hundreds of sailors. In 1497-98, scurvy killed two thirds of Vasco de Gama's men during his voyage to the Indies. The disease continued to kill up to the 18th century, when it was finally learned that it was due to poor diet (lack of vitamin C). But how could a beverage made from pine bark and foliage have cured Jacques Cartier's sailors? This is what Prof. Jacques Masquelier from the University of Bordeaux wanted to find out four centuries later. He left for Quebec in 1950 to learn what was in the pine that saved the sailors from a sure death. He discovered the famous pine OPC's. He would later discover compounds of the same nature in grape peel.

# POLYPHENOLS

# A star molecule of the french paradox: resveratrol

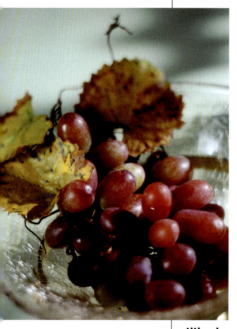

**Polyphenols are excellent weapons in vegetables and resveratrol is one which plays a very important role in explaining the French paradox. It is a natural antibiotic substance produced by plants in response to external elements. It lets the plant defend itself against moulds and bacteria. Resveratrol is present in large quantities in red wine, it primarily accumulates in the grape leaves, peel and seeds. It is one of the stars of the French paradox.**

## It prevents the formation of atheroma.

When a connection was made between drinking wine and the low incidence of cardiovascular diseases despite a diet rich in saturated fats, researchers examined the multiple compounds of red wine. They identified resveratrol as a possible explanation for this phenomenon. It is a compound found in the class of flavonoids. It has a powerful antioxidant action on low-density lipoproteins (the famous LDL or 'bad' cholesterol) and reduces cholesterol deposits on artery walls. It also prevents the formation of atheroma. It is undoubtedly the best cardiovascular protector that can be found in nature. According to the World Health Organization (WHO), resveratrol by itself reduces cardio-vascular risk by 40%.

Resveratrol also prevents platelet sticking, which is responsible for the formation of blood clots. Like drugs such as aspirin, it is also an excellent blood thinner.

## Life expectancy

According to a study conducted by Harvard Medical School, resveratrol activates a longevity gene in certain yeast strains and makes it possible to increase their life expectancy by 70%. Research to date has only involved yeast and flies. Studies are currently in progress on mice. And the good news is that humans possess the same gene.

## Other health benefits

Resveratrol has turned out to have other qualities as well. Thanks to its anti-inflammatory properties, we now know that it is able to assist in preventing the formation and progression of malignant tumours. And it also has a potentially protective action against breast or prostate cancer. Its effectiveness has also been demonstrated in the fight against the spread of fibrous tissues following heart attacks and for treating the flu and certain neurodegenerative diseases.

## A powerful antioxidant

Researchers have incubated human cells with resveratrol and a substance known to produce oxidising lesions. Resveratrol blocked the start of cell death in a dose dependent manner, preventing the damage of the oxidising substance. Researchers concluded that the peripheral blood mononuclear cells acquire an antioxidant power when they are treated with resveratrol.

# The grape, a promise of beauty

Why eat grapes? Because of they sweet, sugary taste, but that's not the only reason. These red fruits represent a real antioxidant cocktail. They contain vitamins, trace elements and polyphenols. In short, the fruit has multiple benefits. Ancient populations knew what they were doing.

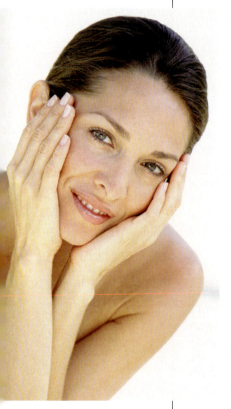

### A concentration of antioxidants

But what does the grape contain that is so exceptional? It is rich in monosaccharides and even more importantly many different vitamins, minerals and trace elements. And of course they contain polyphenols as well. The grape (mainly red) contains a significant quantity of tannins, including the famous OPC's and resveratrol. So why go without it?

### The cosmetic value of OPC's

As well as being powerful free radical receptors, the OPC's contained in grapes are also an excellent defence against ageing. They protect collagen and elastin, the two proteins that create the cohesion and elasticity of our skin and whose alteration results in the appearance of wrinkles. It is also known that these compounds protect against the toxic effects of UV rays, another factor which accelerates skin ageing.

### Eating and drinking grapes

You would have to eat enormous quantities of grapes to get all the benefits for your health.

For example, you would have to drink at least 340 ml of grape juice per day. Researchers estimate that you need to drink three times more grape juice than wine to get the same protective effects. Explanation: most flavonoids are present in the must, a mixture of crushed peel, pulp, seeds and stems. When wine is made, the must is fermented and extracts large quantities of flavonoids which will be present in the wine, while grape juice undergoes only one pressing without fermentation.

## Heart friendly and protector against cancer

Resveratrol, a substance also present in the grape peel, is not only a protector against cardiovascular diseases. It can also contribute to preventing cancer. A study showed that resveratrol effectively prevents three of the stages implicated in the development of skin cancer in mice. Researchers explained this result by the fact that the compound blocks the activity of an enzyme implicated in the onset of cancer.

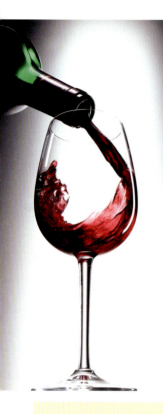

# Wine polyphenols

**Wine polyphenols were long thought to only be important for the colour and aroma of wine. In recent years however, researchers have demonstrated that they are also powerful antioxidants. And as such, that they may be one of the explanations of the French paradox.**

Polyphenols are soluble in wine. This is not the case with those present in most fruits and vegetables. Or, if they are, they do not bind on proteins and thus on the collagen to protect against collagenases. We have also seen that fruit and vegetable polyphenols often end up in the trash with the peels, and even if the entire fruit or vegetable is kept, these compounds often deteriorate with cooking. So in wine, not only is the entire fruit kept, but the wine-making process makes it possible to keep the polyphenols unaltered and to extract a high quantity. This varies with the grape variety, the richest are Pinot Noir, Cabernet Sauvignon and Merlot.

### A phenolic pool

It is not the number of compounds present which makes wine rich in polyphenols, but its diversity and how the polyphenols complement each other. Wine contributes a high quantity of these compounds which are mainly divided into the 6,000 or 7,000 compounds which have been recorded to date. The importance of this breakdown has been particularly demonstrated with the Cretan diet.

### Wine ages... just like us

Bottle ageing of wine is a phenomenon almost as mysterious as human ageing. Like us, a young wine is an acid and turbulent. Then comes the blooming of flavours due

## Too much alcohol... a health risk

In large amounts, alcohol can cause damage to the liver, brain and other organs. The health benefits of alcohol have only been shown with small amounts, so moderation is the key.

## Did you know?

White wines contain ten times fewer polyphenols than red wines. Whites (and rosés) contain between 150 and 600 mg of total polyphenols per litre versus 1500 to 7000 for reds.

to a set of physical-chemical reactions which herald maturity. During this period of its life, wine shows its best side. Before going into a decline, which can be slow or abrupt is based on the origin of the wine.

What are these physical-chemical reactions? When it is put in a cask, the wine is charged with oxygen. And during its ageing, which can last from a year and a half to two years, the phenomenon amplifies. Each year, an average of 20 cm$^3$ of oxygen per litre is dissolved in the wine. After it is bottled, the cork acts as a membrane which distributes oxygen to the wine when it needs it. Don't forget that there are the famous polyphenols which react with the oxygen in the wine. On one side the oxygen and on the other the antioxidants (polyphenols) which continuously do battle resulting in a slow oxidation of the polyphenols. But this phony war actually gives all the aroma and flavour to the wines.

### And alcohol's role in all this?

It is not possible to sing wine's praises without considering the damage caused by alcohol. Comparisons made between Americans and Mediterranean populations show that there is 2 times more breast and colon cancer in the USA compared to the Mediterranean populations. This indicates that if the consumption of alcohol plays a role in these cancers, the Mediterranean diet, including wine, the main alcoholic drink of the Mediterranean, contains compounds which partially neutralize the carcinogenic effect of alcohol.

## Alcohol – How much is too much?

The Dietary Guidelines for Australian's recommend no more than 1 standard drink per day for women and 2 standard drinks a day for men. People with existing health problems or those taking medication should discuss alcohol with their health professional

# Nutritional supplements

**In order to function our body needs essential micronutrients which it cannot synthesise and which it finds in food. But how do we manage to get enough? A healthy well-balanced diet is the first step. However, if your dietary intake is not sufficient, supplements may also be required.**

### Remedy for insufficient intake

Aristotle said: diet is the best medicine. Well he is right, as long as the diet is balanced. The first reason for supplements is based on their definition: a dietary supplement to remedy the insufficiency of daily intake of nutrients.

### Who is at risk?

The changes to the Western diet means that many people may be missing out on essential micronutrients (minerals, vitamins, trace elements and essential fatty acids). If you are at risk for a dietary deficiency, you may require supplements. In particular, those at highest risk include people on a low kilojoules diet, malnourished elderly people, or vegetarians. It is also known that certain circumstances of modern life (overwork, stress, tests, sports, illnesses and ageing) increase our needs for certain nutrients. So, supplements may be the answer. Ask your health professional if you think you may require a supplement.

## Which supplements for what?

1. To fight a polluted environment: all antioxidants
2. To slow the ageing process: all antioxidants
3. For athletes: magnesium, B group vitamins, all antioxidants and iron
4. Skin protection: omega-6, omega-3, ceramides, zinc, selenium, manganese and vitamins C and E.

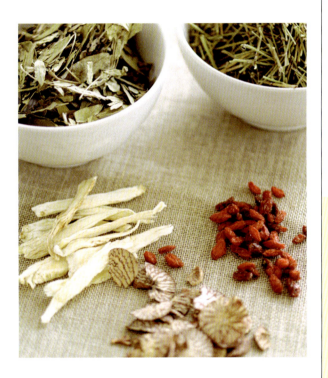

## In plants

Many supplements are plant based. They constitute an extraordinary reserve of antioxidants, and a very wide range exists. Where are they hidden? In wine, tea and chocolate. In ginkgo biloba, olive tree leaves, etc.

These plants can be taken in capsules or teas all year round to reinforce the protection against free radicals, those molecules, which when in excess, contribute to cell deterioration and thus skin ageing, among other things.

## And the quantities?

You need to be cautious. Despite their health benefits, antioxidants and polyphenols should not be consumed in excess. Even if the safe level of intake is unknown, it's important to be aware that too many polyphenols can decrease the absorption of iron. Ask your pharmacist or doctor for advice before taking any supplements.

# The structure and function of skin

**We all care about our skin, this coat that we are born with is a living envelope which protects us from the outside world. Soft and smooth during our first days of life, it fades as time passes and with the various elements it is subjected to. Sun, air pollution, stress and smoking are among its worst enemies. But before examining the processes which causes ageing, let's take a closer look at our skin.**

Seen under a microscope, the skin is composed of three distinct layers: the epidermis, the outermost layer which is a real protective barrier against the outside. The dermis, or intermediate layer, which nourishes and supports the epidermis. And lastly the subcutaneous tissue, a type of fatty mattress, which acts as a shock absorber and more importantly it protects underlying organs.

## Epidermis

Keratinocytes make up 90% of the epidermis. These cells produce keratin, a fibrous protein, which makes the skin impermeable. Keratinocytes constantly renew themselves. Produced in the deepest layer of the epidermis, they flatten themselves and migrant towards the surface where they die. The dead cells form the horny layer, that guards against elements from the outside, with varying degrees of thickness based on the area of our body. Very thin at the level of the eyelids (around fifty microns), the horny layer can reach up to a centimetre at the sole of the foot.

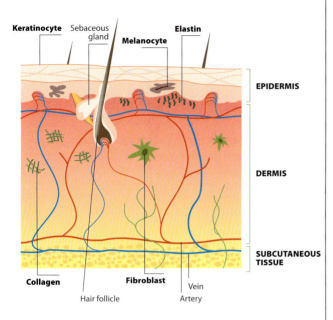

Melanocytes make up the remaining 10% of the epidermis. They produce melanin, a pigment, which helps protects our skin from the sun's rays.

## Dermis

The central layer of the skin is thicker than the epidermis. The dermis is filled with collagen fibres and elastin which give the skin its elasticity and resistance. It contains numerous vessels which nourish the epidermis. The dermis also contains specific nerve endings, sensitive to the touch, pain and heat. This is also where the skin's fluid reserves are found.

## Subcutaneous tissue

It is composed of fatty tissue. It is a type of protective cushion, and is thicker in some parts of the body. In men, this tends to be distributed around the stomach, and in women, the breasts and buttocks.

## Did you know?

The skin is a whole organ, and it is the most important of the human body. In an adult it represents an area of around 1.5 m$^2$ to 2 m$^2$. It weighs between 3.5 and 5 kilos and its thickness varies from 1 to 4 millimetres. It is composed of 2000 billion cells.

# Skin is unique

**Evidence tells us that our ancestors had dark skin (to resist the sun) and were excessively hairy (to protect against temperature changes).**

## Skin Colour

Our skin colour is a simple question of genes. We all possess melanocytes which produce melanin, a natural pigment, controlled by our genes. Depending on its concentration, this pigment makes our epidermis darker or lighter. By the same token, the quantity and intensity of the sun's rays affect our body, which produces more or less melanin to protect itself. This explains all of the variations in skin colour that can be seen travelling around the planet from north to south, from the rosy fair complexions of Nordic populations to the dark skin of Sub-Saharan people.

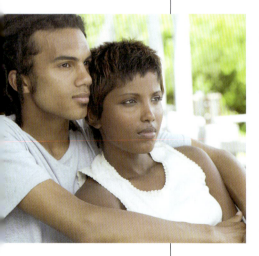

Regardless of skin colour, everyone is born with supple and elastic skin, thanks to collagen and elastin, two structural proteins, present in the dermis of the skin. As we age, the skin starts to show signs of sagging, a consequence of a decrease in the protection of collagen and elastin. And this does not include the action of other external factors, present in our environment (sun, pollution, etc.). However, darker skin is better protected against ageing than fair skin because of the dark melanin, offering better protection from the suns UV rays.

## Skin Types

With a high-powered magnifying glass, any beautician can tell you at a glance whether your skin is normal, dry or oily, or even mixed, a variant of normal skin. Skin type can also influence the rate of ageing.

### - Normal skin

Physiologically, this is skin with a normal moisture level with a horny layer which is not too thin nor too thick and moderate sebaceous secretion. Normal skin does not pull nor peel, it does not turn red, is soft to the touch and can withstand exposure to the elements fairly well. It is the ideal skin. Its variant, mixed skin, is characterized by small pimples, blackheads and a skin which is basically shiny in the middle of the face.

### - Dry skin

Generally fine, this skin type is generally in fluid and fats. So it is more sensitive to external elements, such as sun, pollution, etc. and tends to wrinkle a little quicker.

### - Oily skin

Oily skin is thicker and covered with a layer of water and sebum, this is what gives it its shiny appearance, mainly on the sides of the nose, forehead and chin. Thanks to its hydrolipidic film, oily skin is less sensitive to external factors, and is better able to withstand cold and heat. Stress leaves fewer traces. And so does time

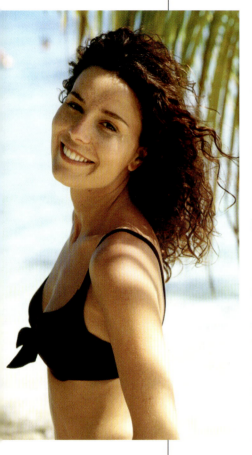

# Functions of the skin

**The skin covers us from head to toe and supports the various parts of our body. It has many functions, the first is to protect us against external elements. Each layer of the skin helps to protect us.**

## Mechanical barrier

The skin protects us against external elements. It acts as a barrier against dust and dirt and anything that can penetrate our body and threaten the tissue and underlying organs. In terms of the epidermis, this role is played by the horny layer. In the dermis, it is assigned to the collagen fibres which give the skin its tautness, and elastin fibres, which put the skin back into place, for example after stretching. Lastly, the small fatty mattresses, which forms the subcutaneous tissue protect against shock and pressure.

## Chemical guard

The skin is a barrier which unfortunately can be penetrated. Certain products can slowly penetrate the skin and later enter the general circulation. In some circumstances this is positive, for example when applying medications. But on the other hand, this can represent a danger, when dealing with toxic products. And babies are more exposed to this danger because their skin is fine and thus more permeable.

## Germ attacks

Our skin's defence against germs is ensured by the horny layer, thanks to its fatty film which acts as a germ barrier. Protection is also provided by the normal bacteria which exists on the skin and fights the development of pathogenic bacteria which cause illnesses. So it's important not to use products which are too aggressive and could destroy the protective bacteria on the skin.

## A sun screen

The skin benefits from the dual protection of the horny layer as well as melanin, which has an increased secretion under the sun. Olive and darks skins, which contain a greater quantity of melanin are thus better protected against the sun than lighter skin.

## Heat regulator

The skin helps keep our body temperature constant. Excess heat is dispersed by dilation of the small vessels in the dermis and through perspiration. When it is cold, on the other hand, the closing of the small vessels, the fatty cushion of the subcutaneous tissue and contraction of small hair muscles help to maintain body heat.

## Babies more exposed to heat stroke

The skin is completely formed at birth, but the secretion of perspiration does not normalise until later. This explains why babies have difficulty regulating their internal temperature and are more exposed to heat stroke.

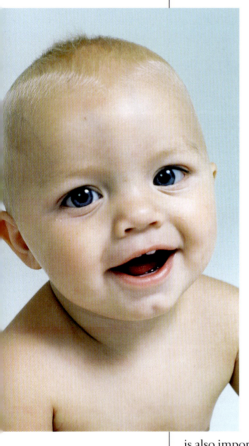

# The skin's best friend

**Collagen makes up 30-35% of the protein in our body. It is by far the most abundant, and is mainly in the skin. Thanks to collagen, we are born with a chubby-cheeked face and firm skin. Unfortunately the production of collagen decreases with age.**

### Chubby cheeks thanks to collagen

Collagen in the skin creates the chubby cheeks seen in babies. We come into this world with an enormous quantity of this protein which compose 90% of the dermis and represents 70% of the weight of young skin. Collagen is made up of three linked polypeptide chains which form a triple helix. These extremely resistant fibres are more solid than steel wires of the same weight. It acts like a cement to give the dermis its solidity and support the epidermis. It is responsible for the firmness and resistance of the skin which can thus better protect against external exposures. Collagen is also important for the scarring process, while the fibres are capable of binding water and thus help moisturise the skin.

This protein is a real gift from the Gods, since it is in such a significant quantity in the skin. As we age, however, the production of collagen decreases and its quality drops, which explains the beginning of wrinkles and changing of the skin. In both men and women the production of collagen starts to decrease at age 20, but this is not apparent right away. The process accelerates from age 40 when the skin becomes drier and finer and loses its radiance.

## An essential protein of connective tissues

Since the three chains can combine in different ways, it is more correct to talk about collagens (plural) than collagen. These proteins are not just found in the skin, but also in the bones, tendons, the cornea and internal organs.

## An essential ingredient!

The word collagen comes from the Greek kolla which means glue. The literal translation of collagen means glue producer. The oldest known glue was made from collagen and dates back 8000 years. The properties of collagen were used by the Egyptians 4000 years ago. Native Americans used it 1500 years ago. It is currently used in beauty products.

## A wire network

The collagen present in the skin makes up a type of wire network which covers the entire thickness of the dermis. The fibre fabric is made of bundles with a molecular mass estimated at 300,000 daltons.

# Ageing:
# Our worst enemy

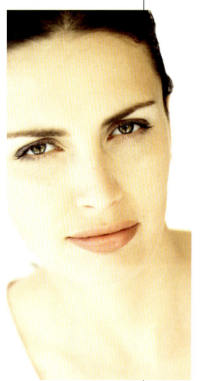

**Ageing is often said to be our worst enemy. One of the causes of ageing is collagenase, an enzyme, which damages the skin.**

Our skin ages like the rest of our body resulting in an increase in number and depth of our wrinkles. These lines are created as a consequence of the deterioration of two dermis proteins, collagen and elastin. The origin of these changes is sometimes biological and sometimes environmental.

The multiplication of oxygenated free radicals (OFR) starts an increase in the activity of certain enzymes implicated in the deterioration of the dermis extracellular matrix. These enzymes are matrix metalloproteinases, of which certain ones, like collagenase cause collagen destruction.

## A poorer synthesis of collagen

The causes of ageing are not well known, but it is believed that it is genetically programmed and affects all organs with a greater sensitivity than organs richer in elastin and collagen, like the lung arteries and the skin. As we age, we produce less dermal keratinocytes and fibroblasts. The consequences of which are a poorer capacity to synthesise collagen. The result being a loose and thin dermis and skin that is not as taut.

## Collagenase almost non-existent in babies

The production of enzymes capable of deteriorating macromolecules, like collagen, increases as we age. While it is relatively weak, or even, nonexistent in young skin or skin protected from the sun. These enzymes start a progressive disruption of the dermis elastic and collagen tissues.

## The fight against ageing and collagenase

The fight against ageing is mainly concentrated on the effects of free radicals. They are hunted down in different ways. This approach is aimed at deflecting the process tied to the overproduction of oxygenated free radicals as well as the over-expression of enzymes, which are a glutton for the skin.

## The virtues of olive oil

Vitamin E (tocophenol) and its by-products contained in olive oil may have a preventative action against skin ageing. This fat soluble vitamin, present in numerous food sources is known to reduce lipid peroxidation. The peroxides which form during skin ageing start an increase in the activity of a protein kinase C associated with the over-expression of collagenase-1. Tocophenol captures the free radicals generated by ageing resulting in a decrease in the production of damaging enzymes.

# Smoking and pollution: accelerators of ageing

**Smoking is very harmful to our health, it increases the risk of cardiovascular diseases, cancers and respiratory diseases. Smoking also has a negative effect on the skin. A dermatologist can tell smokers from non-smokers simply by looking at the appearance of their skin. A smokers complexion is often dull, blotchy and the skin is faded. Wrinkles can appear prematurely on the face.**

It is necessary to remember that the worst pollution is that which is absorbed directly by the body. This is the case with tobacco which is inhaled, resulting in the production of damaging free radicals.

## Nicotine, an ageing agent

The carbon monoxide produced tobacco leaves yellow traces on the fingers, stains the teeth, increases the risk of receding gums, causes dull hair and a decrease in the sizes of the vessels which nourish the skin.

### The skin does not breathe as well

Nicotine and a good appearance don't usually go hand in hand. It is completely the opposite. Tobacco is a scourge for our skin since it has a vasoconstricting effect on blood vessels. When the blood vessels contract they bring less blood and thus less oxygen to our skin cells, which die faster. Tobacco is also a significant source of free radicals, which cause an alteration of the collagen and elastin fibres. To combat the devastating effect of tobacco on the production of these enzymes, an adequate intake of vitamin C is required to stimulates the synthesis of these fibres.

## Smoking gives a gray appearance

The skin of smokers wrinkles faster and becomes more fragile and the complexion can have a gray appearance. The wrinkles and fine lines around the mouth and those around the eyes, the famous expression lines, are much more marked in smokers. Lastly, over time the smoke gets into the pores and blackheads may appear.

## A phenomenon which is can be reversed

The list of the damage that smoke does to our skin does not stop here, but the good news is that this damage is reversible. During the weeks after quitting, the bags under the eyes improve and then disappear, and the complexion brightens. And after six months, the skin is fresher.

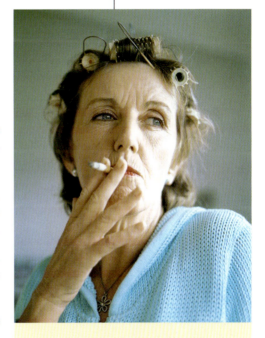

## Women are more exposed

In terms of the skin damage caused by smoking, men and women are not equally affected. Male smokers have more sebum than female smokers, thus their skin is better able to resist the assault of tobacco. This is also true for all the other external elements, such as sun and stress, which our skin is subject to.

# Free radicals

**Free radicals have long been a secret. Until they were recognised as the main causes or ageing, only researchers were interested in them! But what are free radicals? And where do they come from?**

### Our body is the number one source of free radicals

Free radicals are everywhere. Life would be impossible without them. We use them to kill bacteria and viruses and to produce energy. Our body is the main source of free radicals, producing them spontaneously by transforming food into energy through an oxygenation reaction. The problem is that by producing this energy, our cells leave behind free radicals which are pollutants, and toxic waste for our body. Free radical production can increase in certain conditions including pollution, stress, smoking and sun.

### An incomplete chemical formula

Free radicals are a type of chemical which are unstable and very high reactive with neighbouring molecules. Free radicals are capable of oxidising, thus altering proteins, DNA, fatty acids and cell membranes. This is thought to cause ageing with wrinkles appearing due to the hardening of collagen. Not only are free radicals implicated in ageing, they have also been linked to the development of many diseases.

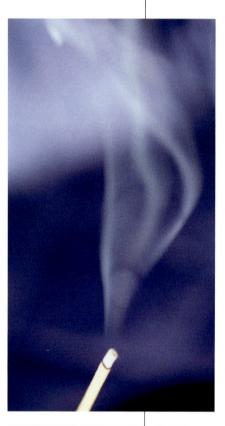

## How does a free radical originate?

We cannot live without oxygen. However, five percent of the oxygen we breathe transforms into a free radical, called superoxide. This is the most common free radical, since it appears every time we burn calories.

## Impressive!

Each year our body naturally produces around 2 kilos of free radicals, and 17 tons over 70 years. A Californian researcher calculated that each of our cells undergoes 10,000 free radical attacks each year.

Fortunately there is an antidote for these toxic poisons: these are the antioxidants which we need more and more as we age. The good news is, nature is filled with these compounds.

### Less free radicals?

It is not possible to produce less free radicals because our body naturally makes what it needs to function. On the other hand, it is possible to act on the external factors which contribute to the production of free radicals. For example, by adopting a healthy lifestyle which eliminates sources of oxidative stress such as smoking, excessive sun, and a high fat diet, we can reduce to production of free radicals.

# CARDIOVASCULAR DISEASES

## Cholesterol: a silent killer

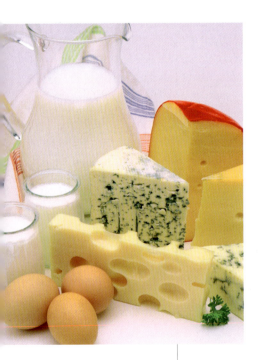

**Cholesterol has been called a silent killer, it acts slowly, discreetly, with serious consequences. High cholesterol is a risk factor for cardiovascular diseases.**

In Australia, an estimated 6 million people have high cholesterol levels. But many ignore this or are not aware and therein lies the danger. Since the damage caused by high cholesterol levels often involves coronary arteries, it can lead to a heart attack. Cholesterol is the most plentiful fatty substance in the animal world and also the most important from a metabolic standpoint. Our bodies need cholesterol to function. This substance has two origins: that supplied by our diet, and that made naturally by the body. The liver is one of the main sites of cholesterol production.

### Present in all cells.

Cholesterol is essential for our body cells. It is a major component of cell membranes. It is also a precursor of steroid hormones  produced by the adrenal glands, ovaries and testicles, and is used by our body, to produce certain substances, including vitamin D. And lastly, cholesterol is an important component of bile.

## Friend or foe?

When there is no excess of cholesterol in our body, there is no problem. As we will see, our body cannot go without it. But it can become a formidable enemy, when there is too much of it.

## Cholesterol: why does it cling to our arteries?

Just like all the other fats, cholesterol is transported throughout the body in the blood stream, by specific molecules called lipoproteins. The low density lipoproteins (LDL) convey it from the liver towards the cells and the high-density lipoproteins (HDL) bring the excess or unused cholesterol to the liver. The LDL has a tendency to accumulate on artery walls. If the LDL level is high, the HDL cannot eliminate it sufficiently. Thus, it is important to distinguish between the two when talking about cholesterol.

## How much fat should be consumed?

Even if you consume good fats, moderation is the key. In a healthy and well-balanced diet, fats should generally make up less than 30% of your daily energy intake.

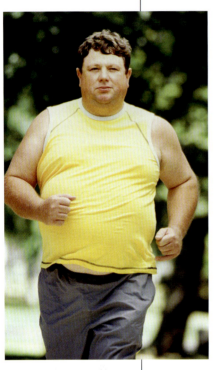

# Good and bad cholesterol

**All epidemiological studies have shown that an excess of bad cholesterol (LDL) and lack of good cholesterol (HDL) represents a cardiovascular risk factor, which can lead to atherosclerosis or hardening of the arteries.**

## HDL-LDL

High-density lipoproteins (HDL) collect the excess cholesterol in the organs and take it to the liver where it is eliminated. In other words, these proteins have the ability to clean all the bad quality fatty deposits from our arteries and also reduce the risk of atheroma.. Thus the name "good" cholesterol.

On the other hand, low-density lipoproteins (LDL) deposit cholesterol on artery walls. Over time, these fats form an accumulation called atheroma which reduces the size of the arteries, making it increasingly difficult for blood to flow, and contributing to the formation of clots. This is why LDL is called bad cholesterol.

## Associated risk factors

For a long time only the total cholesterol level was considered in determining cardiovascular risk. However, the importance of distinguishing between HDL and LDL

## A healthy lifestyle

Lowering your cholesterol level with a balanced diet or when necessary, lipid lowering medication is important, but it may not be enough. You also need to stop smoking (if you smoke), lose weight (if you are overweight) and get regular physical activity. Physical activity is just as important for our body as a good diet.

when looking for cardiovascular risk is now well recognised. This is even more important if you have other risk factors such as high blood pressure, smoking, diabetes, or a family history of heart disease.

## Prevention in the young

All adults, even young adults, should know their cholesterol level. This is because we now know that high cholesterol levels can remain silent for a long time.

## How can you lower your cholesterol level?

Studies have shown that lowering your cholesterol level by 1% results in a double decrease in risk of cardiovascular complications. And an increase of 1% in the HDL (good cholesterol) level decreases this risk by 3%.

### Cholesterol rich foods

While saturated fats have the greatest effect on blood cholesterol levels, the cholesterol found in food can still play a role. The list below describes the cholesterol content of commonly eaten foods. (mg/100g)
- Brains: 1350
- Eggs: 430
- Butter: 230
- Prawns: 150
- Liver: 430

### Food low in cholesterol

Fruits: 0 mg
Vegetables: 0 mg
Cholesterol free margarine: 0 mg
Low fat yoghurt: 0 mg
Skim milk: 0 mg

# Two times fewer cardiovascular events thanks to antioxidants

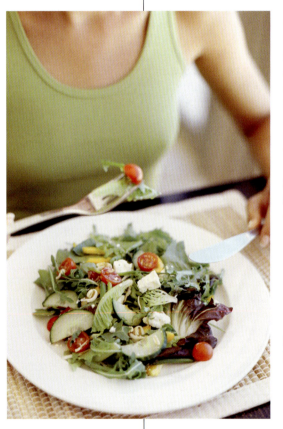

The beneficial effects of dietary intake of antioxidants, micronutrients and polyphenols have mainly been observed in the area of cardiovascular disease prevention. This is hypothesis on which the French paradox is based, and is supported by studies of populations with different diets.

## A leading cause of death in Australia

Cardiovascular diseases are a leading cause of death in Australia, with heart disease reported as the underlying cause of 18% of deaths and stroke causing 8% of deaths. So how can this trend be reversed?

## Antioxidants are good for the heart

Numerous studies suggest that the antioxidants contained in our diet help to prevent cardio vascular diseases. Thus, daily consumption of fruits and vegetables (two serves of fruit and five serves of vegetables per day) decreases the oxyidability of lipoproteins by 30% in smokers. It is also necessary to take the antioxidant power of beverages into account. In particular the consumption of red wine, rich in resveratrol and OPC's (no more than one standard drink a day for women and two standard drinks a day for men) and tea. Some studies have actually shown a relationship between drinking tea and a decrease in the number of heart attacks. Along with the beneficial effects of antioxidants, a diet low in saturated fat and salt (sodium) and high in fibre can help to lower the risk of cardiovascular disease.

## Recommendations

In chapter two (What are antioxidants for?) we mentioned the importance of a pro-antioxidant balance and problems that can occur when there is an imbalance. Nutrition plays a key role in this balance with antioxidants as well as micronutrients (vitamins and trace elements) and polyphenols all playing an important role.

An adequate intake of antioxidants (vitamins, trace elements and polyphenols) are thus essential for reducing the risk of cardiovascular diseases.

Most people who develop heart disease have recognised risk factors. These risk factors include:

Raised cholesterol levels
Raised blood pressure
Smoking
Diabetes
Obesity
Inactivity
Family history of heart disease
Age
Gender

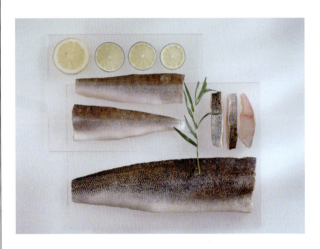

# Omega-3 on the plate

**By now you've probably heard about the health benefits of omega 3's. Omega 3 fats are a 'healthy' fat which our body is unable to make, and must be obtained from our diet.**

Omega-3 is a polyunsaturated fatty acid. Its absorption starts a series of chain reactions, thanks to the help of many enzymes, which contribute to the correct functioning and balance of our body. This is why it is called an essential fatty acid. But our body is not capable of producing it, its only source is from food.

### Our ancestors' plates were full

Our ancestors didn't know whether they were eating omega-3 or how much they were eating. However, their diet was generally filled with it. The first humans who lived around the large African lakes, ate large quantities of fish and shellfish, they also ate game meat which ensured a generous intake of omega-3. Over the centuries, our diet has become increasingly enriched with saturated fats – fast foods are the biggest suppliers. And this is at the expense of these nutritious fatty acids.

## Our heart loves omega 3

Researcher from the University of Laval in Canada discovered the benefits of omega-3 on the cardiac health of the Inuits when compared to the populations of southern Quebec. The latter group, who are heavy smokers, have a diet rich in animal fats and are increasingly obese, however they consume 10 times more fish. Apparently this is what saves them, thanks to the famous omega-3.

## Omega-6 - the balance

Omega-6 is another essential fat which must be balanced with omega 3 to gain optimal health benefits.

# FRUITS AND VEGETABLES THE STARS OF THE FRENCH PARADOX

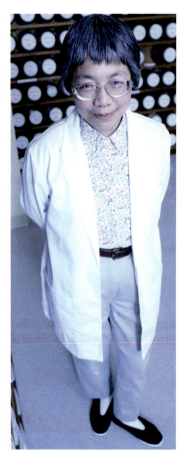

# Answers

**Current nutritional recommendations in Australia, state that for good health Australians need to consume a minimum of 5 serves of vegetables and 2 fruits. That's easy to say. But sometimes not quite as easy to do. Studies have shown that many Australians are not meeting these figures especially for vegetables.**

Moreover, this recommendation is only a minimum. To do this properly, and above all to get real benefits in terms of prevention against cardiovascular diseases, cancer, and other conditions you need to consume a little more than 400 grams of fruit and vegetables. The ideal is between 600-700 grams per day (fresh, canned or frozen). Clearly a large number of people do not achieve this.

### True substance

The pharmaceutical industry has figured out how to get the best from mother nature for our health. From the plant kingdom, it has taken the best, the true substance, in this case the antioxidants which are indispensable for our body to fight the famous free radicals. So, if your diet does not allow you to get all of your antioxidant needs, consider discussing the need for supplements with your health professional.

## An age-old medicine

The manufacturers have not invented anything new. In certain regions of Africa or Central America where doctors are rare but nature flourishes, it is precisely to mother nature that these populations have turned for relief. In these areas where being a healer is passed from generation to generation, plants are an infinitely precious asset. They know all their characteristics and medicinal properties.

## Polyphenol contents and comparitive tables

To be sure to get plenty of antioxidants and namely polyphenols which are wonderful anti-free radicals look for colour. A team from Cirad (international organization for agricultural research for developing countries) measured the quantity of polyphenols in 24 fruits and vegetables. And here are the winners.

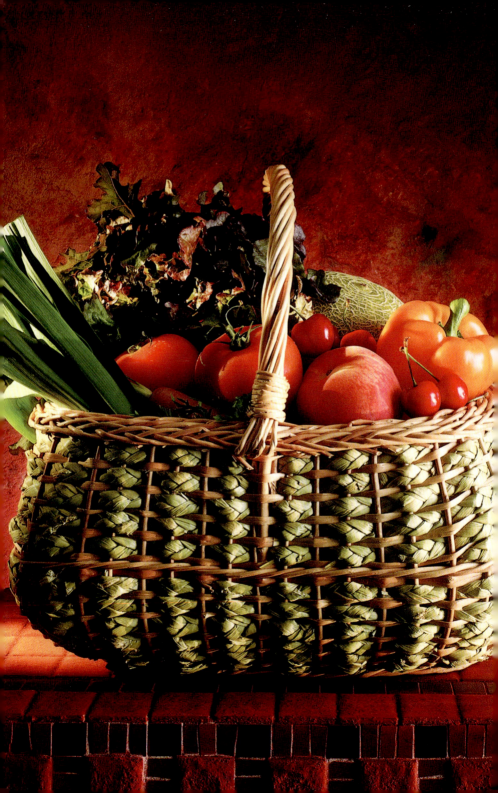

| Rank | Fruit | Total polyphenols (mg GAE / 100g) | Rank | Vegetable | Total polyphenols (mg GAE / 100g) |
|---|---|---|---|---|---|
| 1 | Strawberry | 263.8 | 1 | Artichoke (heart) | 321.3 |
| 2 | Lychee | 222.3 | 2 | Parsley | 280.2 |
| 3 | Grape | 195.5 | 3 | Brussels Sprout | 257.1 |
| 4 | Apricot | 179.8 | 4 | Shallot | 104.1 |
| 5 | Apple | 179.1 | 5 | Broccoli | 98.9 |
| 6 | Date | 99.3 | 6 | Celery | 84.7 |
| 7 | Cherry | 94.3 | 7 | Onion | 76.1 |
| 8 | Fig | 92.5 | 8 | Asparagus | 14.5 |
| 9 | Pear | 69.2 | 9 | Eggplant | 65.6 |
| 10 | White nectarine | 72.7 | 10 | Garlic | 59.4 |
| 11 | Passion fruit | 71.8 | 11 | Turnip | 54.7 |
| 12 | Mango | 68.1 | 12 | Lettuce | 35.6 |
| 13 | Yellow peach | 59.3 | 13 | Celeriac | 39.8 |
| 14 | Banana | 51.5 | 14 | Radish | 38.4 |
| 15 | Pineapple | 47.2 | 15 | Pea | 36.7 |
| 16 | Lemon | 45 | 16 | Leek | 32.7 |
| 17 | Yellow nectarine | 44.2 | 17 | Red pepper | 26.8 |
| 18 | Grapefruit | 43.5 | 18 | Cherry tomato | 26.4 |
| 19 | Orange | 31 | 19 | Potato | 23.1 |
| 20 | Tangerine | 30.6 | 20 | Zucchini | 18.8 |
| 21 | Lime | 30.6 | 21 | Green pepper | 18.2 |
| 22 | Kiwi | 28.1 | 22 | Chicory | 14.7 |
| 23 | Watermelon | 11.6 | 23 | Tomato | 13.7 |
| 24 | Rockmelon | 7.8 | 24 | Fennel | 13 |
| | | | 25 | Cauliflower | 12.5 |
| | | | 26 | Carrot | 10.1 |
| | | | 27 | Green bean | 10 |
| | | | 28 | Avocado | 3.6 |

# Antioxidant beverages

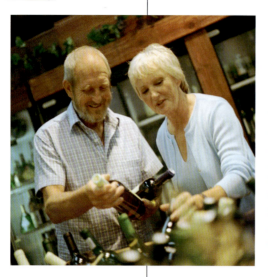

There is no miracle food or drink which can completely erase the effects of ageing on our body. However, there are food and drinks which are richer than others in antioxidant nutrients, these substance protect us against the attacks of free radicals. And we need to place priority on them. This is what the concept of the French paradox is based on.

## What wine tells us

Over the history of humans and their health wine was a privileged beverage. Doctors in the 16th and 18th century talked about wines "to strengthen youth" which helped with digestion and increased natural warmth, preventing or healing diseases such as the plague. But there was also the flip side of the coin: the same doctors also talked about wine clouding the senses and causing headaches. Wine continued to be the subject of debate in the 20th and 21st centuries. But the French paradox theory established its fame in scientific circles.

## Tea and wine protect against oxidizing damage

Tea, wine and cocoa all have a high polyphenol content from the family of flavonoids which are sources of antioxidants certainly less known than fruits and vegetables, but not less interesting. Recent experimental

### The cranberry

This small red berry grows primarily in the bogs in the eastern part of the United States and Canada.. Rich in polyphenols, it has been mainly of interest in the prevention of urinary tract infections.

studies have established that flavonoids derived from red wine and tea can be absorbed by the intestine and detected in the plasma where they play an important role in the protection against the oxidizing damage of LDL. The may also reduce the growth of atheroma which is the first lesion of cardiovascular disease.

The best known flavonoids in tea are the catechins which have an antioxidizing activity 4 times higher than vitamins E or C.

## Contents in polyphenols (mg per cup)

Red wine: 340
Green tea: 165
Black tea: 124

## Colours to protect against the sun

Generally foods and beverages which have a high quantity of pigments or polyphenols can have a protective action against the sun. This is the case of tea, red wine, grapes, raspberries, currents and cranberries. The flavonoids they contain are powerful antioxidants.

**In our collection Alpen Éditions:**

-The Omega-3 Answer

-Living with a Hyperactive Child

-All About the Prostate

-The French Paradox

-The XXL Syndrome

**with Michel Montignac:**

-Eat Yourself Slim

-The Montignac Diet Cookbook

-The French GI Diet

-Glycemic Index Diet

**www.alpen.mc**